HEMOCHROMATOSIS COOKBOOK

80+ Easy Wholesome Recipes to Reduce
Iron Absorption and Fight Iron Overload

SCARLETT LAWSON

CONTENT

BREAKFAST & BRUNCH

SALAD

VEGETABLE

DESSERT & BEVERAGE

BREAKFAST & BRUNCH

TURMERIC HERB EGG SALAD

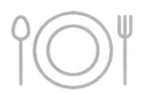

PREP TIME	COOK TIME	SERVES
5 MINUTES	NA	4

INGREDENTS

8 hard boiled eggs, peeled and mashed

1 cup chopped mixed herbs such as parsley, dill, tarragon or chives

1 cup chopped onion

1/2 cup chopped celery

1/3 cup plain low fat yogurt

1 tablespoon mayonnaise

1 tablespoon apple cider vinegar

3/4 teaspoon turmeric

1/4 teaspoon salt

DIRECTIONS

1. In a large bowl, combine all ingredients.

THIS RECIPE CONTAINS:

√ CALCIUM   √ POLYPHENOLS

√ CURCUMIN   √ *Bioflavonoids*

√ LACTOFERRIN   √ *Phenolic acids*

√ PECTIN   *Tannins*

  PHYTATES   √OXALATES

√ PHOSVITIN

BREAKFAST & BRUNCH

SMOKEY YOGURT DEVILED EGGS

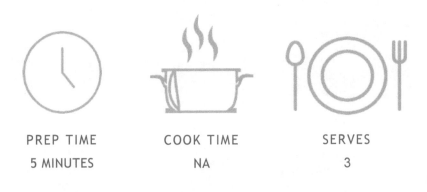

PREP TIME	COOK TIME	SERVES
5 MINUTES	NA	3

INGREDENTS

6 hard boiled eggs, peeled and halved

3/4 cup low fat Greek yogurt

2 tablespoons sun-dried tomatoes, finely chopped

3/4 teaspoon smoked paprika

1/4 teaspoon salt

DIRECTIONS

1. Scoop out the egg yolks into a medium bowl. Combine with yogurt, sun-dried tomatoes, paprika and salt.

2. Scoop the mixture back into the egg white and serve.

THIS RECIPE CONTAINS:

√ CALCIUM

CURCUMIN

√ LACTOFERRIN

√ PECTIN

PHYTATES

√ PHOSVITIN

POLYPHENOLS

Bioflavonoids

Phenolic acids

Tannins

OXALATES

BREAKFAST & BRUNCH

2-MINUTE COFFEE MUG CAKE

PREP TIME
5 MINUTES

COOK TIME
2 MINUTES

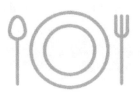

SERVES
1

INGREDENTS

1 large egg,

3 tablespoons strong brewed coffee

2 tablespoons coconut flour

1 1/2 tablespoons maple syrup

1 tablespoon chopped pecans

1/4 teaspoon baking powder

1/4 teaspoon cinnamon

1/4 teaspoon vanilla extract

Pinch of salt

DIRECTIONS

1. Combine all ingredients in a large mug.

2. Microwave for 90 seconds. Use a toothpick to check if the center is cooked through. Microwave for an extra 30 seconds if needed.

THIS RECIPE CONTAINS:

CALCIUM	√ POLYPHENOLS
CURCUMIN	√ *Bioflavonoids*
LACTOFERRIN	√ *Phenolic acids*
PECTIN	√ *Tannins*
√ PHYTATES	OXALATES
√ PHOSVITIN	

BREAKFAST & BRUNCH

BEET AND QUINOA BREAKFAST BOWL

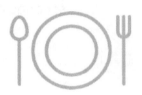

PREP TIME
5 MINUTES

COOK TIME
5 MINUTES

SERVES
1

INGREDENTS

1 cup cooked quinoa

1 small beet, finely grated

1 cup full fat milk

1/4 cup mixed berries

1 tablespoon honey

1 tablespoon chopped almonds

1 tablespoon chopped walnuts

1 teaspoon cinnamon

1/4 teaspoon vanilla extract

DIRECTIONS

1. Combine all ingredients and serve.

THIS RECIPE CONTAINS:

√ CALCIUM

CURCUMIN

√ LACTOFERRIN

PECTIN

√ PHYTATES

PHOSVITIN

√ POLYPHENOLS

√ *Bioflavonoids*

√ *Phenolic acids*

Tannins

√ OXALATES

BREAKFAST & BRUNCH

SPINACH SALMON PEAS OMELET

PREP TIME
5 MINUTES

COOK TIME
5 MINUTES

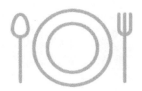

SERVES
1

INGREDENTS

2 large eggs, beaten

1 5-ounce can pink salmon, drained and flaked

1/2 cup frozen peas, thawed

1/2 cup baby spinach, chopped

2 tablespoons grated cheddar cheese

1 tablespoon coconut oil

salt and pepper to taste

DIRECTIONS

1. Boil the peas for 2 minutes. Drain and set aside.

2. In a pan, add oil and sauté spinach until wilted. Add eggs. Season with salt and pepper. Cover and cook for 1-2 minutes or until egg is almost set. Remove from heat.

3. Add peas, salmon and cheese then fold in half. Return to the heat and cook for another 1-2 minutes or until the cheese has melted.

THIS RECIPE CONTAINS:

√ CALCIUM

CURCUMIN

√ LACTOFERRIN

√ PECTIN

√ PHYTATES

√ PHOSVITIN

√ POLYPHENOLS

√ *Bioflavonoids*

√ *Phenolic acids*

Tannins

√ OXALATES

BREAKFAST & BRUNCH

TURMERIC SCRAMBLED EGGS

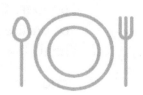

PREP TIME	COOK TIME	SERVES
5 MINUTES	10 MINUTES	2

INGREDENTS

4 large eggs

3 cups fresh baby spinach

3 tablespoons half and half

1 tablespoon chopped fresh parsley

1 teaspoon turmeric

1 teaspoon coconut oil

Pinch of salt

DIRECTIONS

1. In a pan, add the oil and sauté spinach and cook until wilted.

2. Meanwhile, combine the rest of the ingredients in a bowl.

3. Add the egg mixture to the pan and keep stirring until it reaches desired consistency.

4. Top with chopped parsley and serve.

THIS RECIPE CONTAINS:

√ CALCIUM   √ POLYPHENOLS

√ CURCUMIN   √ *Bioflavonoids*

√ LACTOFERRIN   √ *Phenolic acids*

PECTIN   *Tannins*

PHYTATES   √ OXALATES

√ PHOSVITIN

BREAKFAST & BRUNCH

VEGETABLE FRITTATA

PREP TIME
5 MINUTES

COOK TIME
15 MINUTES

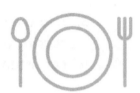

SERVES
4

INGREDENTS

8 large eggs, beaten

1/2 medium onion, chopped

1/2 bell pepper, chopped

2 cups chopped fresh kale

2 cups chopped fresh spinach

1 1/2 cups chopped mushrooms

1/2 cup half and half

1/2 cup grated parmesan cheese

1 tablespoon minced fresh parsley

1 tablespoon minced fresh basil

1 tablespoon coconut oil

salt to taste

DIRECTIONS

1. Preheat the oven to 375 °F.

2. In a pan, add oil and sauté onion, bell peppers and mushrooms until fragrant. Transfer to a bowl and then sauté kale and spinach until wilted. Remove excess water.

3. In a medium bowl, combine herbs, half and half and eggs. Season with salt.

THIS RECIPE CONTAINS:

√ CALCIUM

CURCUMIN

√ LACTOFERRIN

√ PECTIN

PHYTATES

√ PHOSVITIN

√ POLYPHENOLS

√ *Bioflavonoids*

√ *Phenolic acids*

Tannins

√ OXALATES

BREAKFAST & BRUNCH

SPICY TOMATOES SCRAMBLED EGGS

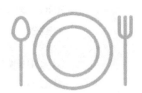

PREP TIME	COOK TIME	SERVES
5 MINUTES	15 MINUTES	2

INGREDENTS

4 large eggs. Beaten

1 large tomato, seeded and chopped

1/2 medium onion, chopped

1/4 cup half and half

2 tablespoons coconut oil

1 tablespoons chopped fresh parsley

1/2 teaspoon smoked paprika

1/4 teaspoon oregano

salt and pepper to taste

DIRECTIONS

1. In a medium bowl, combine eggs and half and half. Season with salt and pepper.

2. In a pan, add oil and sauté onion with paprika and oregano until fragrant. Add tomatoes and cook until fragrant.

3. Add the egg mixture to the pan and keep stirring until it reaches desired consistency.

4. Top with chopped parsley and serve.

THIS RECIPE CONTAINS:

√ CALCIUM   √ POLYPHENOLS

CURCUMIN   √ Bioflavonoids

√ LACTOFERRIN   √ Phenolic acids

√ PECTIN   Tannins

PHYTATES   √ OXALATES

√ PHOSVITIN

BREAKFAST & BRUNCH

PIZZA FRITTATA

PREP TIME
5 MINUTES

COOK TIME
15 MINUTES

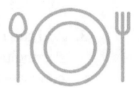

SERVES
2

INGREDENTS

3 large eggs, beaten

1/2 medium onion, sliced

2 cloves garlic, minced

1 cup shredded mozzarella cheese

1/2 cup sliced mushrooms

1/4 cup tomato sauce

3 tablespoons milk

2 tablespoons coconut oil

salt and pepper to taste

DIRECTIONS

1. Preheat the broiler

2. In a pan, add oil and sauté onion, mushroom and garlic until fragrant. Remove excess water. Season with salt and pepper.

3. In a small bowl, combine eggs with milk.

4. Add in egg mixture. Cover and cook on medium for 2-3 minutes until the egg is set. Transfer to a pie dish.

5. Spread the tomato sauce and sprinkle the mozzarella cheese on top. Broil for 3-5 minutes or until the cheese melted.

THIS RECIPE CONTAINS:

√ CALCIUM   √ POLYPHENOLS

CURCUMIN   *Bioflavonoids*

√ LACTOFERRIN   √ *Phenolic acids*

√ PECTIN   *Tannins*

PHYTATES   √ OXALATES

√ PHOSVITIN

BREAKFAST & BRUNCH

WALNUT CRANBERRY MUFFINS

PREP TIME
15 MINUTES

COOK TIME
25 MINUTES

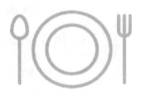

SERVES
12

INGREDENTS

4 large eggs, separated

1 large very ripe banana, peeled and mashed

1 cup fresh cranberry

1/2 cup walnuts, chopped

1 cup blanched almond flour

1/3 cup coconut flour

1/2 cup full fat milk

1/2 cup coconut oil, melted

2 teaspoons vanilla extract

2 teaspoons baking powder

1 teaspoon ground ginger

1/4 teaspoon salt

DIRECTIONS

1. Preheat the oven to 350 °F.

2. In a medium bowl, combine coconut oil, banana, egg yolks, coconut milk and vanilla extract.

3. In another bowl, mix almond flour, coconut flour, baking powder, salt and ginger.

4. In a mixing bowl, beat the egg whites until they form soft peaks.

5. Add flour mixture to banana mixture in batches and mix until well combined. Then gently fold half of the egg white into the mixture. Add cranberry and chopped walnut before folding in the rest of the egg whites.

6. Divide the mixture into 12 muffin cups. Bake for 20-25 minutes or until the center is set.

THIS RECIPE CONTAINS:

√ CALCIUM   √ POLYPHENOLS

CURCUMIN   √ Bioflavonoids

√ LACTOFERRIN   √ Phenolic acids

PECTIN   Tannins

√ PHYTATES   √ OXALATES

√ PHOSVITIN

BREAKFAST & BRUNCH

CARROT TURMERIC MUFFINS

PREP TIME
15 MINUTES

COOK TIME
25 MINUTES

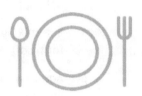

SERVES
12

INGREDENTS

3 large eggs, separated

1 cup grated carrot

1/2 cup shredded coconut

2 cups blanched almond flour

1/2 cup coconut oil

1/2 cup maple syrup

1 tablespoon grated fresh ginger

1 teaspoon baking soda

1/2 teaspoon turmeric

1/2 teaspoon cinnamon

pinch of clove

DIRECTIONS

1. Preheat the oven to 350 °F.

2. In a medium bowl, combine coconut oil, maple syrup and egg yolks.

3. In another bowl, mix almond flour, shredded coconut, baking soda, salt and spices.

4. In a mixing bowl, beat the egg whites until they form soft peaks.

5. Add flour mixture to oil mixture in batches and mix until well combined. Then gently fold half of the egg white into the mixture. Add grated carrot and grated ginger before folding in the rest of the egg whites.

6. Divide the mixture into 12 muffin cups. Bake for 20-25 minutes or until the center is set.

THIS RECIPE CONTAINS:

√ CALCIUM

√ CURCUMIN

LACTOFERRIN

√ PECTIN

√ PHYTATES

√ PHOSVITIN

√ POLYPHENOLS

Bioflavonoids

√ Phenolic acids

Tannins

√ OXALATES

BREAKFAST & BRUNCH

PUMPKIN CHIA SEED MUFFINS

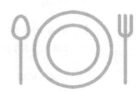

PREP TIME	COOK TIME	SERVES
15 MINUTES	25 MINUTES	12

INGREDENTS

6 large eggs, separated

1 cup pumpkin puree

1 1/2 cups almond flour

1/2 cup coconut oil, melted

1/2 cup maple syrup

1/4 cup ground chia seed

1/3 pumpkin seeds

1 tablespoon pumpkin pie mix

1 teaspoon baking powder

1/2 teaspoon salt

DIRECTIONS

1. Preheat the oven to 350 °F.

2. In a medium bowl, combine coconut oil, pumpkin puree, maple syrup and egg yolks.

3. In another bowl, mix almond flour, chia seeds, baking powder, salt and spices.

4. In a mixing bowl, beat the egg whites until they form soft peaks.

5. Add flour mixture to oil mixture in batches and mix until well combined. Then gently fold the egg white into the mixture in batches.

6. Divide the mixture into 12 muffin cups. Top with pumpkin seeds. Bake for 20-25 minutes or until the center is set.

THIS RECIPE CONTAINS:

√ CALCIUM   √ POLYPHENOLS

CURCUMIN   *Bioflavonoids*

LACTOFERRIN   √ *Phenolic acids*

√ PECTIN   *Tannins*

√ PHYTATES   √ OXALATES

√ PHOSVITIN

BREAKFAST & BRUNCH

EASY STUFFED TOMATOES

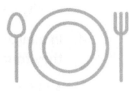

PREP TIME
20 MINUTES

COOK TIME
20 MINUTES

SERVES
2

INGREDENTS

2 medium tomatoes, flesh scooped out and set side

1/3 cup leftover quinoa or rice

1/2 small carrot, peeled and roughly chopped

1/2 rib celery, roughly chopped

1/2 small onion, peeled and roughly chopped

1 clove garlic, peeled

2 tablespoons coconut oil

2 tablespoons grated parmesan cheese

1 tablespoon chicken broth

1 tablespoon chopped fresh basil

1 teaspoon turmeric

1/4 teaspoon dried oregano

salt and pepper to taste

DIRECTIONS

1. Preheat the oven to 375 °F.

2. Use a food processor or blender, blend the scooped out tomatoes, carrot, celery, onion and garlic into rice-size pieces.

3. In a pan, add oil an sauté the veggie with turmeric and oregano until fragrant.

4. Add broth and simmer uncovered for 2-3 minutes. Stir in quinoa, cheese and basil. Season with salt and pepper. Remove from heat.

5. Stuff the tomato and Bake for 15-20 minutes until heated through.

THIS RECIPE CONTAINS:

√ CALCIUM	√ POLYPHENOLS
√ CURCUMIN	√ Bioflavonoids
√ LACTOFERRIN	√ Phenolic acids
√ PECTIN	Tannins
√ PHYTATES	√OXALATES
PHOSVITIN	

BREAKFAST & BRUNCH

MULTISEED BREAKFAST MUFFINS

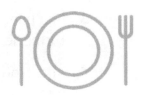

PREP TIME	COOK TIME	SERVES
15 MINUTES	25 MINUTES	12

INGREDENTS

6 large eggs, beaten

1 cup almond meal

1/2 cup ground hemp seed

1/2 cup cottage cheese

1/2 cup grated parmesan cheese

1/4 cup chopped green onion

1/4 cup flax seed meal

1/2 teaspoon baking powder

1/2 teaspoon paprika

1/2 teaspoon turmeric

1/4 teaspoon salt

DIRECTIONS

1. Preheat the oven to 375 °F.

2. In a mixing bowl, combine almond meal, hemp seed, parmesan cheese, flaxseed meal, baking powder, spices and salt.

3. In another bowl, combine cottage cheese and eggs until smooth. Add the mixture to the dry ingredients. Mix until well combined.

THIS RECIPE CONTAINS:

√ CALCIUM

√ CURCUMIN

√ LACTOFERRIN

PECTIN

√ PHYTATES

PHOSVITIN

√ POLYPHENOLS

√ *Bioflavonoids*

√ *Phenolic acids*

Tannins

√ OXALATES

BREAKFAST & BRUNCH

CHEESY CAULIFLOWER QUESADILLAS

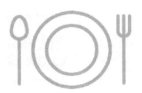

PREP TIME	COOK TIME	SERVES
20 MINUTES	20 MINUTES	6

INGREDENTS

1 large head Cauliflower, florets only

3 large eggs

1 1/2 cup shredded cheddar cheese

3/4 cup shredded mozzarella cheese

6 tablespoons mayonnaise

2 tablespoons coconut oil

3/4 teaspoon paprika

1/2 teaspoon turmeric

1/2 teaspoon sea salt

1/2 teaspoon xanthan gum

DIRECTIONS

1. Preheat the oven to 400 °F.
2. Use a food processor, pulse the cauliflower into rice-size pieces. Transfer to a bowl and microwave on high until cooked, about 8-10 minutes. Set aside to cool.
3. Use a cheese cloth to squeeze out excess water.
4. Use the food processor with the S blade, combine cauliflower rice, eggs, mozzarella cheese, turmeric and salt until smooth. Sprinkle xanthan gum bit by bit and blend until smooth.
5. Pour the mixture into 6 portions on a baking sheet and spread using a spoon. Bake for 8-10 minutes before flipping. Bake for another 4-6 minutes. Remove from oven and let it cool for 10 minutes.
6. Meanwhile. In a small bowl, mix mayonnaise with paprika.
7. Once the tortilla is cooled enough, spread 1 tablespoon on sauce, top with cheddar cheese and fold in half.
8. In a pan, add oil and fry the quesadillas for 2-3 minutes per side.

THIS RECIPE CONTAINS:

√ CALCIUM   POLYPHENOLS

√ CURCUMIN   Bioflavonoids

√ LACTOFERRIN   Phenolic acids

PECTIN   Tannins

PHYTATES   OXALATES

√ PHOSVITIN

BREAKFAST & BRUNCH

SMOKED LENTIL CHEESE BURGERS

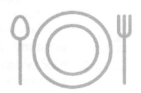

PREP TIME	COOK TIME	SERVES
5 MINUTES	45 MINUTES	6

INGREDENTS

1 cup red lentils

1 large egg

1/4 medium onion, finely chopped

1/4 cup grated cheddar cheese

1 tablespoon coconut oil

1/2 teaspoon ground coriander

1/2 teaspoon turmeric

1/2 teaspoon smoked paprika

1/4 teaspoon salt

1/4 teaspoon pepper

DIRECTIONS

1. Boil lentils in 2 cups of water for 25 minutes. Drain.

2. In a mixing bowl, combine all ingredients except oil. Shape the mixture into burgers.

3. In a pan, add oil and cook the burger over medium-high heat for 5 minutes per side or until golden brown

THIS RECIPE CONTAINS:

√ CALCIUM

√ CURCUMIN

√ LACTOFERRIN

√ PECTIN

√ PHYTATES

√ PHOSVITIN

√ POLYPHENOLS

√ *Bioflavonoids*

√ *Phenolic acids*

Tannins

√ OXALATES

BREAKFAST & BRUNCH

SOUTHWEST EGG MUFFINS

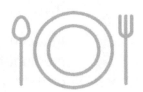

PREP TIME	COOK TIME	SERVES
5 MINUTES	45 MINUTES	6

INGREDENTS

6 large eggs, beaten

1 large red bell pepper, seeded and chopped

1 4-ounce can diced green chilis, drained

2 green onions, chopped

1/2 cup grated mexican blend cheese

1/4 cup sour cream

1 tablespoon coconut oil

1/2 teaspoon paprika

salt and pepper to taste

DIRECTIONS

1. Preheat the oven to 375 °F.

2. In a pan, add oil and sauté bell peppers and green chilis until fragrant. Then divide the mixture into 6 muffin cup, followed by green onions and cheese.

3. In a large measuring cup, whisk the sour cream until soften. All beaten eggs and paprika. Mix until well combined. Pour over the cups evenly. Bake for 25-30 minutes or until center is set.

THIS RECIPE CONTAINS:

√ CALCIUM

CURCUMIN

√ LACTOFERRIN

PECTIN

PHYTATES

√ PHOSVITIN

√ POLYPHENOLS

Bioflavonoids

√ *Phenolic acids*

Tannins

OXALATES

BREAKFAST & BRUNCH

SAVORY SUPERFOOD BOWL

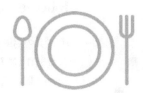

PREP TIME	COOK TIME	SERVES
30 MINUTES	30 MINUTES	4

INGREDENTS

4 kale leaves, washed and roughly chopped

1 avocado, seeded and sliced

1 15-ounce can chickpeas, rinsed and drained

1/2 cup quinoa

2 tablespoons roasted sesame seeds

1 tablespoon coconut oil

2 teaspoons turmeric

1 teaspoon smoked paprika

pinch of salt

DIRECTIONS

1. Preheat the oven to 350 °F.

2. Coat the chickpeas in paprika and lay evenly on a baking sheet. Drizzle with coconut oil and season with salt. Bake for 25 minutes.

3. Meanwhile, boil the quinoa with 1 cup of water for about 20 minutes. Drain well and mix with turmeric.

4. In each serving bowl, add kale leaves, 1/4 of avocado, chickpeas and quinoa. Top with sesame seed before serving.

THIS RECIPE CONTAINS:

√ CALCIUM   √ POLYPHENOLS

√ CURCUMIN   √ *Bioflavonoids*

LACTOFERRIN   √ *Phenolic acids*

√ PECTIN   *Tannins*

√ PHYTATES   √ OXALATES

PHOSVITIN

BREAKFAST & BRUNCH

KALE FETA CASSEROLE

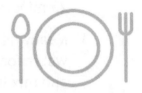

PREP TIME
5 MINUTES

COOK TIME
55 MINUTES

SERVES
8

INGREDENTS

12 ounces kale, washed and roughly chopped

12 large eggs, beaten

3/4 cup crumbled feta cheese

2 teaspoons coconut oil

1 teaspoon smoked paprika

1 teaspoon turmeric

Salt and pepper to taste

DIRECTIONS

1. Preheat the oven to 375 °F.

2. sauté kale and cook until wilted. Transfer to a greased casserole dish. Top with crumbled feta cheese.

3. Add the spices and seasoning to the beaten eggs. Pour the egg on top. Bake for 40-45 minutes.

THIS RECIPE CONTAINS:

√ CALCIUM

√ CURCUMIN

√ LACTOFERRIN

PECTIN

PHYTATES

√ PHOSVITIN

√ POLYPHENOLS

Bioflavonoids

√ *Phenolic acids*

Tannins

√ OXALATES

BREAKFAST & BRUNCH

PARMESAN FRIED EGGPLANTS

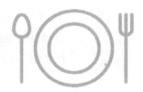

PREP TIME
30 MINUTES

COOK TIME
30 MINUTES

SERVES
6

INGREDENTS

1 medium Eggplant, sliced into 1/3" thick slices

1 large egg, beaten

1 cup almond flour

1 cup grated parmesan cheese

1/4 cup coconut oil

1/2 teaspoon salt

1/2 teaspoon pepper

DIRECTIONS

1. Line the eggplant slices on a baking sheet. Sprinkle with salt and let it sit for half an hour. Use paper towels to remove excess moisture.

2. In a plate, mix almond flour, parmesan, salt and pepper.

3. In a pan, heat 2 tablespoons of coconut oil. Dip each eggplant slices in egg mixture then flour mixture. Shake off excess flour before frying. Fry for 3-5 minutes per side or until golden brown. Repeat with the rest of the slices.

THIS RECIPE CONTAINS:

√ CALCIUM

CURCUMIN

√ LACTOFERRIN

√ PECTIN

√ PHYTATES

√ PHOSVITIN

√ POLYPHENOLS

√ *Bioflavonoids*

√ *Phenolic acids*

Tannins

√ OXALATES

BREAKFAST & BRUNCH

CHEESY SPINACH PIE

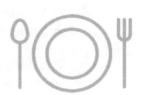

PREP TIME	COOK TIME	SERVES
15 MINUTES	55 MINUTES	12

INGREDENTS

Crust:

1 1/2 cups almond flour

1 tablespoon coconut flour

1 egg

salt and pepper to taste

Filling:

1 pound frozen spinach, thawed and squeezed dry

5 large eggs, beaten

1/2 onion, finely chopped

8 ounces cream cheese

8 ounces crumbled feta cheese

salt and pepper to taste

DIRECTIONS

1. Preheat the oven to 350 °F.

2. In a medium bowl, combine all crust ingredients. Grease a 9" pie dish. Add the crust mixture and press into firm crust with a glass. Poke a few times with a fork.

3. Bake for 15 minutes.

4. Meanwhile, Combine all filling ingredients. Add to the dish after the crust is baked.

5. Bake for another 40 minutes or until center is set.

THIS RECIPE CONTAINS:

√ CALCIUM   √ POLYPHENOLS

CURCUMIN   √ *Bioflavonoids*

√ LACTOFERRIN   √ *Phenolic acids*

PECTIN   *Tannins*

PHYTATES   √ OXALATES

√ PHOSVITIN

BREAKFAST & BRUNCH

SPINACH ZUCCHINI LASAGNA

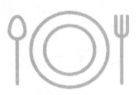

PREP TIME	COOK TIME	SERVES
20 MINUTES	50 MINUTES	9

INGREDENTS

4 medium zucchini, sliced lengthwise into 1/8" thick slices

1/2 medium onion, finely chopped

4 cloves garlic, minced

1 28-ounce crushed tomatoes

1 pound ricotta cheese

1 pound shredded mozzarella cheese

3 cups spinach

1/4 cup grated parmesan cheese

2 tablespoons tomato paste

1 tablespoon coconut oil

1 tablespoon chopped fresh basil

salt and pepper to taste

DIRECTIONS

1. Preheat the broiler

2. In a pan, add oil and sauté onion and garlic until fragrant. Add tomato paste and crushed tomatoes. Season with salt. Bring to a boil and reduce to low heat. Simmer for 25-30 minutes. Remove from heat and stir in spinach and basil.

3. Line the zucchini on a baking sheet and broil for 5-8 minutes. Remove from oven and let it cool. Then remove excess moisture with paper towels.

4. In a bowl, combine egg, ricotta cheese and parmesan cheese.

5. In a greased 9" x 12' casserole dish, start with tomato sauce, then add a layer of zucchini, followed by egg/cheese mixture then mozzarella cheese. Repeat the layers. Top the final layer with sauce and mozzarella.

6. Bake covered for 30 minutes then 10 minutes uncovered. Let it sit for 15 minutes before serving.

THIS RECIPE CONTAINS:

√ CALCIUM	√ POLYPHENOLS
CURCUMIN	√ *Bioflavonoids*
√ LACTOFERRIN	√ *Phenolic acids*
√ PECTIN	*Tannins*
PHYTATES	√ OXALATES
√ PHOSVITIN	

BREAKFAST & BRUNCH

MATCHA ALMOND LOAF CAKE

PREP TIME
15 MINUTES

COOK TIME
60 MINUTES

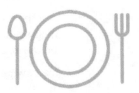

SERVES
12

INGREDENTS

3 large eggs, separated

3 1/2 cups almond flour

1/2 cup coconut oil, melted

1/2 cup maple syrup

2 tablespoons hot water

1 tablespoon Matcha green tea powder

1 1/2 teaspoon baking powder

1 teaspoon baking soda

1/2 teaspoon salt

DIRECTIONS

1. Preheat the oven to 300 °F.

2. Dissolve the Matcha powder in hot water.

3. In a medium bowl, mix almond flour, baking powder, baking soda and salt.

4. In another bowl, mix coconut oil, egg yolks, maple syrup.

5. In a mixing bowl, beat the egg whites until they form soft peaks.

6. Add flour mixture to oil mixture in batches and mix until well combined. Then gently fold the egg white into the mixture in batches.

7. Add the batter into a loaf pan. Bake for 60 minutes or until center is set.

THIS RECIPE CONTAINS:

√ CALCIUM

CURCUMIN

LACTOFERRIN

PECTIN

√ PHYTATES

√ PHOSVITIN

√ POLYPHENOLS

√ *Bioflavonoids*

√ *Phenolic acids*

√ *Tannins*

√ OXALATES

BREAKFAST & BRUNCH

GINGERBREAD CHIA PUDDING

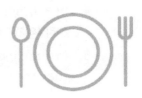

PREP TIME	COOK TIME	SERVES
8 HOURS	NA	1

INGREDENTS

1/4 cup chia seeds

3/4 cup full fat milk

1 tablespoon honey or maple syrup

1 tablespoon chopped pecans or almonds

1/4 teaspoon ground ginger

1/2 teaspoon cinnamon

pinch of salt

DIRECTIONS

1. Combine all ingredients except chopped nuts in a mason jar. Refrigerate overnight.

2. Top with nuts and serve.

THIS RECIPE CONTAINS:

√ CALCIUM

CURCUMIN

√ LACTOFERRIN

PECTIN

√ PHYTATES

PHOSVITIN

√ POLYPHENOLS

√ *Bioflavonoids*

√ *Phenolic acids*

Tannins

√ OXALATES

SALAD

KALE APPLE ALMOND SALAD

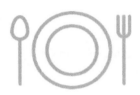

PREP TIME	COOK TIME	SERVES
5 MINUTES	NA	4

INGREDENTS

For the Salad:

4 cups finely chopped kale

2 tablespoons chopped almonds

1 medium apple, diced

1/4 cup shredded cheddar cheese

2 tablespoons shredded parmesan cheese

For the Dressing:

1/4 cup avocado oil

2 tablespoons lemon juice

1 clove garlic, minced

Salt and pepper to taste

DIRECTIONS

1. In a small bowl, whisk all dressing ingredients until well combined.

2. Toss the dressing with the salad and serve.

THIS RECIPE CONTAINS:

√ CALCIUM

CURCUMIN

√ LACTOFERRIN

√ PECTIN

√ PHYTATES

PHOSVITIN

√ POLYPHENOLS

√ *Bioflavonoids*

√ *Phenolic acids*

Tannins

√ OXALATES

SALAD

BLACK BEAN AND LENTIL SALAD

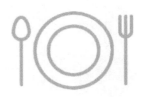

PREP TIME
5 MINUTES

COOK TIME
NA

SERVES
4

INGREDENTS

For the Salad:

2 cups cooked lentils

1 15-ounce can black beans, rinsed and drained

2 medium tomatoes, chopped

1/2 medium red onion, sliced

8 ounces crumbled goat cheese

1 cup chopped fresh cilantro

For the Dressing:

1 lime, juice only

2 tablespoons avocado oil

1 teaspoon Dijon mustard

2 cloves garlic, minced

1/2 teaspoon oregano

salt and pepper to taste

DIRECTIONS

1. In a small bowl, whisk all dressing ingredients until well combined.

2. Toss the dressing with the salad and serve.

THIS RECIPE CONTAINS:

√ CALCIUM

CURCUMIN

√ LACTOFERRIN

PECTIN

√ PHYTATES

PHOSVITIN

√ POLYPHENOLS

√ *Bioflavonoids*

√ *Phenolic acids*

Tannins

√ OXALATES

SALAD

CHICKPEAS FETA BEAN SALAD

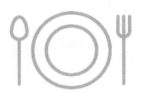

PREP TIME	COOK TIME	SERVES
5 MINUTES	NA	4

INGREDENTS

For the Salad:

1 15-ounce can chickpeas, rinsed and drained

1 15-ounce can red kidney beans, rinsed and drained

1 medium red onion, diced

4 scallions, green part only, chopped

1 cup chopped fresh parsley

1/2 cup crumbled feta cheese

For the Dressing:

1 lemon, juice only

1 tablespoon avocado oil

2 cloves garlic, minced

1 tablespoons grated fresh ginger

salt and pepper to taste

DIRECTIONS

1. In a small bowl, whisk all dressing ingredients until well combined.

2. Toss the dressing with the salad and serve.

THIS RECIPE CONTAINS:

√ CALCIUM

CURCUMIN

√ LACTOFERRIN

PECTIN

√ PHYTATES

PHOSVITIN

√ POLYPHENOLS

√ Bioflavonoids

√ Phenolic acids

Tannins

√ OXALATES

SALAD

CURRY CHICKEN SALAD

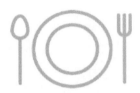

PREP TIME
5 MINUTES

COOK TIME
NA

SERVES
2

INGREDENTS

For the Salad:

1 1/2 cup cooked and shredded chicken

1 stalk celery, chopped

1 medium cucumber, chopped

For the Dressing:

1/3 cup mayonnaise

1 teaspoon curry powder

1/4 teaspoon turmeric

salt and pepper to taste

DIRECTIONS

1. In a small bowl, whisk all dressing ingredients until well combined.

2. Toss the dressing with the salad and serve.

THIS RECIPE CONTAINS:

CALCIUM	√ POLYPHENOLS
√ CURCUMIN	√ *Bioflavonoids*
LACTOFERRIN	√ *Phenolic acids*
√ PECTIN	*Tannins*
PHYTATES	OXALATES
PHOSVITIN	

SALAD

TURMERIC KALE AND QUINOA SALAD

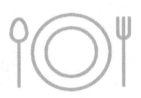

PREP TIME	COOK TIME	SERVES
5 MINUTES	NA	4

INGREDENTS

For the Salad:

4 cups chopped kale

2 cups cooked quinoa

3 scallions, green parts only, chopped

1/4 cup chopped almonds

For the Dressing:

1/4 cup avocado oil

1/2 lemon, juice only

2 tablespoons honey

1 teaspoon turmeric

salt and pepper to taste

DIRECTIONS

1. In a small bowl, whisk all dressing ingredients until well combined.

2. Toss the dressing with the salad and serve.

THIS RECIPE CONTAINS:

CALCIUM	√ POLYPHENOLS
√ CURCUMIN	√ Bioflavonoids
LACTOFERRIN	√ Phenolic acids
PECTIN	Tannins
√ PHYTATES	√ OXALATES
PHOSVITIN	

SALAD

CRANBERRY SPINACH SALAD

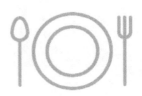

PREP TIME	COOK TIME	SERVES
5 MINUTES	NA	4

INGREDENTS

For the Salad:

5 cups baby spinach

1/2 cup dried cranberries

2 tablespoons toasted
sesame seeds

For the Dressing:

1/4 cup avocado oil

2 tablespoons apple cider
vinegar

2 tablespoons honey or
maple syrup

2 cloves garlic, minced

1/4 teaspoon smoked
paprika

DIRECTIONS

1. In a small bowl, whisk all dressing ingredients until well combined.

2. Toss the dressing with the salad and serve.

THIS RECIPE CONTAINS:

CALCIUM

CURCUMIN

LACTOFERRIN

PECTIN

√ PHYTATES

PHOSVITIN

√ POLYPHENOLS

√ *Bioflavonoids*

√ *Phenolic acids*

Tannins

√ OXALATES

SALAD

POMEGRANATE WILD RICE SALAD

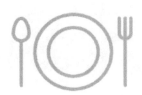

PREP TIME	COOK TIME	SERVES
5 MINUTES	NA	4

INGREDENTS

For the Salad:

3 cups cooked wild rice

5 cups chopped arugula

1 pomegranate, seeds only

4 ounces crumbled feta cheese

1/2 cup chopped walnuts

For the Dressing:

6 tablespoons avocado oil

2 tablespoons apple cider vinegar

1 teaspoon honey or maple syrup

1 clove garlic, minced

salt and pepper to taste

DIRECTIONS

1. In a small bowl, whisk all dressing ingredients until well combined.

2. Toss the dressing with the salad and serve.

THIS RECIPE CONTAINS:

√ CALCIUM

CURCUMIN

√ LACTOFERRIN

√ PECTIN

√ PHYTATES

PHOSVITIN

√ POLYPHENOLS

√ *Bioflavonoids*

√ *Phenolic acids*

Tannins

OXALATES

SALAD

QUICK CARROT SLAW

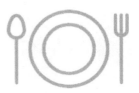

PREP TIME	COOK TIME	SERVES
10 MINUTES	NA	4

INGREDENTS

4 large carrots, peeled and shredded

1 lemon, juice only

1/4 cup sesame oil

1/4 cup coconut amino

3 tablespoons sesame seed

1/2 teaspoon ground ginger

1/2 teaspoon turmeric

DIRECTIONS

1. In a mixing bowl, toss all ingredients together. Adjust seasoning if needed.

THIS RECIPE CONTAINS:

CALCIUM	√ POLYPHENOLS
√ CURCUMIN	√ *Bioflavonoids*
LACTOFERRIN	√ *Phenolic acids*
√ PECTIN	*Tannins*
√ PHYTATES	√ OXALATES
PHOSVITIN	

SALAD

CREAMY CUCUMBER DILL SALAD

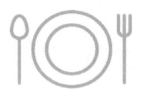

PREP TIME
10 MINUTES

COOK TIME
NA

SERVES
2

INGREDENTS

1 large cucumber, shredded

1/3 cup sour cream

2 tablespoons chopped fresh dill

1 tablespoon apple cider vinegar

2 teaspoons raw honey or maple syrup

salt and pepper to taste

DIRECTIONS

1. In a small bowl, whisk all ingredients except cucumber until well combined.

2. Toss the dressing with cucumber and serve.

THIS RECIPE CONTAINS:

√ CALCIUM

CURCUMIN

√ LACTOFERRIN

√ PECTIN

PHYTATES

PHOSVITIN

√ POLYPHENOLS

√ *Bioflavonoids*

√ *Phenolic acids*

Tannins

OXALATES

SALAD

AVOCADO GREEK SALAD

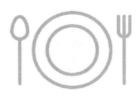

PREP TIME	COOK TIME	SERVES
10 MINUTES	NA	2

INGREDENTS

For the Salad:

1 medium cucumber, shredded

2 medium tomatoes, chopped

1/2 medium red onion, sliced

1 medium avocado, seeded and diced

For the Dressing:

2 tablespoons avocado oil

1 tablespoon apple cider vinegar

1 garlic, minced

1 teaspoon oregano

Pinch of salt

DIRECTIONS

1. In a small bowl, whisk all dressing ingredients until well combined.

2. Toss the dressing with the salad and serve.

THIS RECIPE CONTAINS:

√ CALCIUM

CURCUMIN

√ LACTOFERRIN

√ PECTIN

PHYTATES

PHOSVITIN

√ POLYPHENOLS

√ *Bioflavonoids*

√ *Phenolic acids*

Tannins

√ OXALATES

SALAD

ZUCCHINI WALNUT SALAD

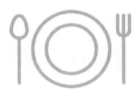

PREP TIME	COOK TIME	SERVES
10 MINUTES	10 MINUTES	2

INGREDENTS

1 Zucchini, seeded and cut into half moons

1/2 head romaine lettuce

1/3 cup chopped walnuts

1/3 cup shredded parmesan cheese

2 tablespoons chopped scallion

For the Dressing:

1/3 cup mayonnaise

1 teaspoon lemon juice

1 clove garlic, minced

1/4 teaspoon salt

Pinch of pepper

DIRECTIONS

1. In a pan, add avocado oil and sauté zucchini until slightly brown. Season with salt and pepper. Transfer to a large mixing bowl. Add the rest of the vegetables.

2. Add walnuts to the pan and roast for a few minutes. Season with salt and pepper. Transfer to the mixing bowl.

3. In a small bowl, combine all dressing ingredients. Toss with the salad, top with cheese and serve.

THIS RECIPE CONTAINS:

√ CALCIUM

CURCUMIN

√ LACTOFERRIN

PECTIN

√ PHYTATES

√ PHOSVITIN

√ POLYPHENOLS

√ *Bioflavonoids*

√ *Phenolic acids*

Tannins

√ OXALATES

SALAD

CRANBERRIES BROCCOLI SALAD

PREP TIME
15 MINUTES

COOK TIME
5 MINUTES

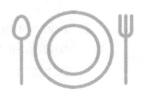

SERVES
4

INGREDENTS

For the Salad:

1 large head broccoli, florets only

2 stalks celery, finely chopped

3 tablespoons chopped dried cranberries

1/4 red onion, finely chopped

For the Dressing:

2 tablespoons Greek yogurt

2 tablespoons mayonnaise

2 tablespoons lemon juice

1 teaspoon Dijon mustard

1/2 teaspoon turmeric

1/2 teaspoon salt

Pinch of ground black pepper

DIRECTIONS

1. In a small bowl, whisk all dressing ingredients until well combined.

2. Toss the dressing with the salad and serve.

THIS RECIPE CONTAINS:

√ CALCIUM

CURCUMIN

√ LACTOFERRIN

√ PECTIN

PHYTATES

PHOSVITIN

√ POLYPHENOLS

√ Bioflavonoids

√ Phenolic acids

Tannins

√ OXALATES

SALAD

CARROT LENTIL SALAD

PREP TIME
10 MINUTES

COOK TIME
20 MINUTES

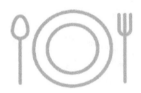

SERVES
4

INGREDENTS

1 cup dry lentil

1 large carrot, peeled and diced

1 medium red onion, chopped

1 stalk celery, chopped

2 cloves garlic, minced

1 bay leaf

1/4 cup chopped fresh parsley

1/4 cup avocado oil

1/2 teaspoon thyme

2 tablespoons lemon juice

salt and pepper to taste

DIRECTIONS

1. In a pan, add lentils carrots, garlic, bay leaf and thyme. Add water over 1 inch and simmer until lentils are cooked, about 20 minutes. Remove bay leave and drain.

2. In a mixing bowl, mix the cooked ingredients with the rest of the ingredients and serve.

THIS RECIPE CONTAINS:

CALCIUM

CURCUMIN

LACTOFERRIN

√ PECTIN

√ PHYTATES

PHOSVITIN

√ POLYPHENOLS

√ Bioflavonoids

√ Phenolic acids

Tannins

√ OXALATES

SALAD

ROASTED BEET CARROT SALAD

PREP TIME
10 MINUTES

COOK TIME
40 MINUTES

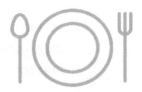

SERVES
2

INGREDENTS

For roasted beet and carrot:

4 medium beetroots, peeled and cut into 1 1/2"-chunks

2 medium carrots, peeled and cut into 1 1/2"-chunks

1 1/2 tablespoons avocado oil or coconut oil

1 teaspoon minced fresh thyme

3/4 teaspoon salt

1/2 teaspoon ground black pepper

For Salad:

1 medium cucumber, sliced

1 medium red onion, sliced

1/2 head red leaf lettuce, sliced

8 ounces feta cheese, crumbled

For dressing:

1/3 cup avocado oil

1/4 cup lemon juice

salt and pepper to taste

DIRECTIONS

1. Preheat the oven to 400 °F.

2. Toss the beetroots and carrots with oil, thyme, salt and pepper. Roast for 35-40 minutes or until tender, turning once half way through.

3. Transfer roasted beet and carrots with the rest of the salad ingredients and serve.

THIS RECIPE CONTAINS:

√ CALCIUM

CURCUMIN

√ LACTOFERRIN

√ PECTIN

PHYTATES

PHOSVITIN

√ POLYPHENOLS

√ *Bioflavonoids*

√ *Phenolic acids*

Tannins

√ OXALATES

SALAD

ROASTED TOMATOES CAPRESE

PREP TIME
10 MINUTES

COOK TIME
2 HOURS

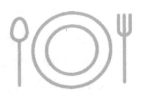

SERVES
2

INGREDENTS

4 plum tomatoes, seeded and halved

6 ounces fresh salted mozzarella, cut into 1/2"- slices

4 fresh basil leaves, julienned

1 1/2 tablespoons avocado oil

1/2 tablespoon balsamic vinegar

1 clove garlic, minced

1 teaspoon maple syrup

1/2 teaspoon salt

1/4 teaspoon ground black pepper

DIRECTIONS

1. Preheat the oven to 275 °F.

2. Toss the tomatoes with oil and vinegar. Drizzle with syrup and sprinkle with salt and pepper. Bake for 2 hours. Allow to cool.

3. Line the tomatoes and mozzarella alternatively. Season with ground black pepper. Top with basil and serve

THIS RECIPE CONTAINS:

√ CALCIUM   √ POLYPHENOLS

CURCUMIN   √ *Bioflavonoids*

√ LACTOFERRIN   √ *Phenolic acids*

√ PECTIN   *Tannins*

PHYTATES   √ OXALATES

PHOSVITIN

VEGETABLE

VEGGIE RICE PAPER ROLL WITH
SPICY PEANUT SAUCE

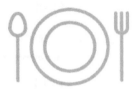

PREP TIME	COOK TIME	SERVES
30 MINUTES	NA	2

INGREDENTS

For the rolls:

8 sheets rice paper

1 cup shredded red cabbages

1 cup julienned carrots

1 cup julienned cucumbers

1 large red bell pepper, thinly sliced

1 large yellow bell pepper , thinly sliced

1 cup fresh cilantro leaves

For the sauce:

1 cup roasted salted peanuts

1 clove garlic, chopped

1/4 cup avocado oil

1/4 cup soy sauce or coconut amino

1/4 cup fresh lime juice

3 tablespoons sesame oil

1 1/2 tablespoons maple syrup

1 1/2 tablespoons hot sauce or to taste

DIRECTIONS

1. Use a food processor to pulse all sauce ingredients into desired consistency.

2. Soak the rice paper in cold water for 15 seconds. Place a small handful of each vegetables. Roll up tightly.

3. Repeat with the rest of the ingredients.

THIS RECIPE CONTAINS:

CALCIUM

CURCUMIN

LACTOFERRIN

√ PECTIN

√ PHYTATES

PHOSVITIN

√ POLYPHENOLS

√ Bioflavonoids

√ Phenolic acids

Tannins

√ OXALATES

VEGETABLE

RATATOUILLE STEW

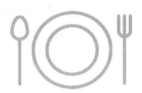

PREP TIME
5 MINUTES

COOK TIME
25 MINUTES

SERVES
4

INGREDENTS

1 8-ounce can crushed tomatoes

1 medium red bell pepper, chopped

4 cloves garlic, minced

1/2 medium onion, chopped

2 cups chopped eggplants

1 small zucchini, chopped

1 cup vegetable broth

1/4 cup chopped fresh basil

1/4 cup shredded cheddar cheese

2 tablespoons toasted pine nuts

1 tablespoon avocado oil

salt and pepper to taste

DIRECTIONS

1. In a pan, add oil and sauté garlic, onion and bell pepper until fragrant.

2. Add eggplant, zucchini and broth. Simmer for 15 minutes or until vegetables are tender.

3. Stir in crushed tomatoes. Season with salt and pepper.

4. Top with cheese and pine nuts before serving.

THIS RECIPE CONTAINS:

√ CALCIUM	√ POLYPHENOLS
CURCUMIN	√ Bioflavonoids
√ LACTOFERRIN	√ Phenolic acids
√ PECTIN	Tannins
√ PHYTATES	√ OXALATES
PHOSVITIN	

VEGETABLE

QUICK SUPERBEANS CHILI

PREP TIME
10 MINUTES

COOK TIME
20 MINUTES

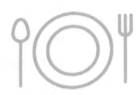

SERVES
4

INGREDENTS

1 15-ounce can kidney beans, rinsed and drained

1 15-ounce black beans, rinsed and drained

1 15-ounce can diced tomatoes

1 medium red bell pepper, diced

1 medium onion, diced

4 cloves garlic, minced

2 cups vegetable broth

3/4 cup tomato paste

1/2 cup soup cream

2 tablespoons chili pepper (optional)

1 tablespoon avocado oil

1 teaspoon smoked paprika

1 teaspoon oregano

salt to taste

DIRECTIONS

1. In a pan, add oil and sauté garlic, onion, bell pepper and all seasoning until fragrant.

2. Add the rest of the ingredients except sour cream. Simmer for 10-15 minutes or until thickened.

3. Top with sour cream and serve.

THIS RECIPE CONTAINS:

√ CALCIUM

CURCUMIN

√ LACTOFERRIN

√ PECTIN

√ PHYTATES

PHOSVITIN

√ POLYPHENOLS

√ Bioflavonoids

√ Phenolic acids

Tannins

√ OXALATES

VEGETABLE

CHEESY TURMERIC BROCCOLI SOUP

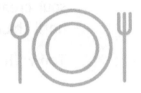

PREP TIME
20 MINUTES

COOK TIME
20 MINUTES

SERVES
4

INGREDENTS

1 cup chopped broccoli florets

1 medium onion, diced

2 cloves garlic, minced

2 cups vegetable broth

1 cup cheddar cheese

1/4 cup heavy cream

1/4 cup chopped pecans

2 tablespoons coconut oil

1/2 teaspoon turmeric

salt and pepper to taste

DIRECTIONS

1. In a pan, sauté onion and garlic until fragrant.

2. Add broth, turmeric and broccoli. Cook until tender. Season with salt and pepper.

3. Stir in heavy cream, bring to a boil and remove from heat.

4. Stir in cheddar cheese. Top with chopped pecans and serve.

THIS RECIPE CONTAINS:

√ CALCIUM

√ CURCUMIN

√ LACTOFERRIN

√ PECTIN

√ PHYTATES

PHOSVITIN

√ POLYPHENOLS

√ Bioflavonoids

√ Phenolic acids

Tannins

√ OXALATES

VEGETABLE

QUINOA STUFFED ZUCCHINI BOAT

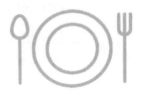

PREP TIME
15 MINUTES

COOK TIME
35 MINUTES

SERVES
4

INGREDENTS

4 small zucchini, halved and seed removed

1/4 cup grated mozzarella cheese

For filling:

1 cup cooked quinoa

1/2 cup baby spinach, chopped

4 ounces cream cheese

1 tablespoon chopped fresh basil

1/2 teaspoon oregano

salt and pepper to taste

DIRECTIONS

1. Preheat the oven to 375 °F.

2. In a large bowl, combine all filling ingredients. Season with salt and pepper.

3. Divide the mixture in the zucchini halves. Bake for 30-35 minutes uncovered. Top with mozzarella and bake for another 10 minutes.

THIS RECIPE CONTAINS:

√ CALCIUM   √ POLYPHENOLS

CURCUMIN   √ *Bioflavonoids*

√ LACTOFERRIN   √ *Phenolic acids*

√ PECTIN   *Tannins*

√ PHYTATES   √ OXALATES

PHOSVITIN

VEGETABLE
TOMATO SOUP WITH
CHICKPEAS CROUTONS

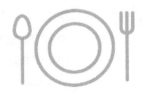

PREP TIME
10 MINUTES

COOK TIME
40 MINUTES

SERVES
4

INGREDENTS

For the soup:

1 28-ounce can whole peeled tomatoes, with juice

1 medium onion, diced

2 cloves garlic, minced

1 1/2 cup vegetable broth

1/2 cup heavy cream

1/4 cup oil-pack sun-dried tomatoes

1/4 cup tomato paste

1 tablespoon coconut oil

1 teaspoon dried oregano

salt and pepper to taste

For Croutons:

1 15-ounce chickpeas, rinsed ,drained and dried

1 teaspoon coconut oil, melted

1/2 teaspoon fried oregano

1/2 teaspoon turmeric

1/2 teaspoon salt

DIRECTIONS

1. Preheat the oven to 425 °F.

2. Toss chickpeas with oil and seasoning and line on a baking sheet. Bake for 25-30 minutes or until golden, turning once half way through. Set aside to cool.

3. Meanwhile, in a pan, sauté onion and garlic until fragrant. Transfer to a food processor.

4. Add the rest of the soup ingredients except cream and blend until smooth.

5. When the chickpeas are almost done, return the soup to the sauce pan. Heat and stir in cream.

6. Top with the chickpeas croutons and serve.

THIS RECIPE CONTAINS:

√ CALCIUM	√ POLYPHENOLS
√ CURCUMIN	√ *Bioflavonoids*
√ LACTOFERRIN	√ *Phenolic acids*
√ PECTIN	*Tannins*
√ PHYTATES	√ OXALATES
PHOSVITIN	

VEGETABLE

TURMERIC PUMPKIN SOUP

PREP TIME
10 MINUTES

COOK TIME
40 MINUTES

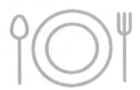

SERVES
4

INGREDENTS

1 medium butternut squash, seeded and cut into chunks

1 cup coconut milk

1/2 cup half and half

1/4 cup chopped walnuts

1 large onion, diced

3 cloves garlic, peeled

1 1/2 tablespoons grated fresh ginger

1 tablespoon coconut oil

1 1/2 teaspoon turmeric

3 sage leaves

salt and pepper to taste

DIRECTIONS

1. Preheat the oven to 350 °F.

2. Toss the squash in oil. Season with salt and pepper. Bake for 40 minutes. Add onion and garlic half way through.

3. Use a food processor or blender to blend the roasted vegetables and the rest of the ingredients except walnuts until smooth.

4. Heat the soup in a sauce pan. Top with chopped walnut and serve.

THIS RECIPE CONTAINS:

√ CALCIUM

CURCUMIN

√ LACTOFERRIN

√ PECTIN

√ PHYTATES

PHOSVITIN

√ POLYPHENOLS

√ Bioflavonoids

√ Phenolic acids

Tannins

√ OXALATES

VEGETABLE

CAULIFLOWER PESTO PIZZA

PREP TIME
20 MINUTES

COOK TIME
40 MINUTES

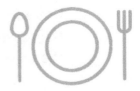

SERVES
6

INGREDENTS

For the Crust:

2 medium heads cauliflowers, florets only

2 large eggs, whites only

4 cloves garlic, minced

1 1/2 cups grated parmesan cheese

1 teaspoon Italian seasoning

For the Sauce:

1/2 cup Plain Greek Yogurt

1/2 cup packed fresh basil

2 cloves garlic

1 tablespoon avocado oil

salt and pepper to taste

For topping:

2 cooked skinless chicken breast, shredded

2 plum tomatoes, sliced

1/2 cup grated parmesan cheese

2 tablespoons chopped fresh basil

94

DIRECTIONS

1. Preheat the oven to 400 °F.

2. Use a food processor, pulse the cauliflower into rice-size pieces. Transfer to a bowl and microwave on high until cooked, about 8-10 minutes. Set aside to cool.

3. Use a cheese cloth to squeeze out excess water. Transfer to a large mixing ball.

4. Combine cauliflower with egg whites, garlic, Italian seasoning and cheese. Mold into 4 mini-pizza crust or 1 large pizza crust. Bake for 30 minutes.

5. Meanwhile, use a food processor to blend all the pesto sauce ingredients. Adjust seasoning if needed.

6. After the crust is cooked, change to broiler setting.

7. Spread the sauce on the pizza(s). Top with tomato slices and chicken. Season with salt and pepper. Top with parmesan and broil for 3-5 minutes until cheese turns golden. Sprinkle with basil and serve.

THIS RECIPE CONTAINS:

√ CALCIUM   √ POLYPHENOLS

CURCUMIN   √ *Bioflavonoids*

√ LACTOFERRIN   √ *Phenolic acids*

√ PECTIN   *Tannins*

PHYTATES   √ OXALATES

√ PHOSVITIN

LEGUMES & GRAINS

QUINOA SUSHI ROLL

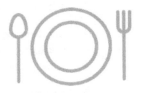

PREP TIME
10 MINUTES

COOK TIME
NA

SERVES
1

INGREDENTS

2 nori sheet

1/2 cup cooked quinoa

1/4 avocado, sliced

1 small cucumber, thinly sliced

1 small carrot, julienned

1 small beetroot, grated

Soy sauce and wasabi to serve (optional)

DIRECTIONS

1. **Place the nori sheet on a flat counter. Spread half the rice on the sheet, leaving about 1-inch at the top and moisten the edge with water**

2. **Line half of each ingredients near the bottom of the sheet.**

3. **Tightly roll up and serve with soy sauce and wasabi.**

THIS RECIPE CONTAINS:

√ CALCIUM   √ POLYPHENOLS

CURCUMIN   √ *Bioflavonoids*

LACTOFERRIN   √ *Phenolic acids*

√ PECTIN   *Tannins*

√ PHYTATES   √ OXALATES

PHOSVITIN

LEGUMES & GRAINS

GOLDEN QUINOA FRIED "RICE"

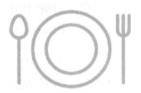

PREP TIME	COOK TIME	SERVES
5 MINUTES	15 MINUTES	4

INGREDENTS

3 cups leftover quinoa

2 medium carrots, diced

4 shallots, chopped

2 eggs, beaten

2 cloves garlic, minced

1/2 onion, diced

1/2 cup frozen peas, thawed

2 tablespoons soy sauce/coconut amino

3 tablespoons sesame oil,

1 teaspoon paprika

1 teaspoon coriander

1/2 teaspoon turmeric

1/2 teaspoon ground ginger

DIRECTIONS

1. In a pan, add 1 tablespoon of sesame oil and scramble the egg until cooked. Set aside.

2. Add the rest of the oil and sauté shallots, garlic, onion, carrot, peas and all the spices until vegetables soften.

3. Add quinoa and soy sauce/coconut amino. Stir fry until heat thoroughly. Return the egg and mix well. Serve immediately.

THIS RECIPE CONTAINS:

CALCIUM	√ POLYPHENOLS
√ CURCUMIN	√ *Bioflavonoids*
LACTOFERRIN	√ *Phenolic acids*
√ PECTIN	*Tannins*
√ PHYTATES	√ OXALATES
√ PHOSVITIN	

LEGUMES & GRAINS

SPICY TOMATO FRIED RICE

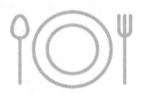

PREP TIME	COOK TIME	SERVES
5 MINUTES	15 MINUTES	4

INGREDENTS

2 cups leftover brown rice

1 medium onion, diced

1/2 lime, juice only

2/3 cup fire roasted tomatoes

1/4 cup chopped fresh cilantro

1 tablespoon coconut oil

1 tablespoon tomato paste

1 teaspoon minced pickled jalapeños

1 teaspoon chili powder or to taste

1/2 teaspoon smoked paprika

salt and pepper to taste

DIRECTIONS

1. In a pan, add oil and sauté onion until fragrant. Add tomatoes, tomato paste and all seasoning. Cook for 1-2 minutes.

2. Add rice and lime juice. Stir fry until heated thoroughly. Garnish with fresh cilantro and serve.

THIS RECIPE CONTAINS:

CALCIUM

CURCUMIN

LACTOFERRIN

√ PECTIN

√ PHYTATES

PHOSVITIN

√ POLYPHENOLS

√ Bioflavonoids

√ Phenolic acids

Tannins

√ OXALATES

LEGUMES & GRAINS

PUMPKIN QUINOA BOWL

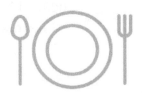

PREP TIME
15 MINUTES

COOK TIME
15 MINUTES

SERVES
2

INGREDENTS

1 cup cooked quinoa

1/2 small pumpkin, seeded and cut into small chunks

1 stalk celery, sliced

1/4 cup dried cranberry

1/4 cup chopped pecans

1 tablespoon butter

salt and pepper to taste

For the dressing:

1/3 cup Greek yogurt

1/4 cup Italian blue cheese

2 tablespoons milk

DIRECTIONS

1. In a small bowl, combine the dressing ingredients. Refrigerate.

2. In a pan, sauté pumpkin with butter and oil until tender. Add celery and cranberries and cook for another 5 minutes. Season with salt and pepper.

3. In a large bowl, mix the sautéed vegetables with cooked quinoa. Top with yogurt dressing and serve.

THIS RECIPE CONTAINS:

√ CALCIUM

CURCUMIN

√ LACTOFERRIN

√ PECTIN

√ PHYTATES

PHOSVITIN

√ POLYPHENOLS

√ *Bioflavonoids*

√ *Phenolic acids*

Tannins

√ OXALATES

LEGUMES & GRAINS

TURMERIC LENTILS SPINACH DAAL

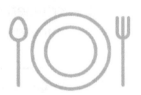

PREP TIME	COOK TIME	SERVES
5 MINUTES	25 MINUTES	2

INGREDENTS

1/2 cup red lentils

4 cups baby spinach

1 red chili, finely chopped

1/2 medium onion, chopped

3/4 cup water

3/4 cup plain yogurt

1 vegetable stock cube, crumbled

2 tablespoons chopped fresh cilantro

1 tablespoon coconut oil

1 tablespoon fresh lemon juice

1 teaspoon turmeric

salt and pepper to taste

DIRECTIONS

1. In a pan, add oil and sauté chili and onion with turmeric and stock cube until fragrant.

2. Add lentils and stir fry for 1 minute. Add half of the water and cook until the liquid is absorbed.

3. Add spinach and the rest of the liquid. Cook until spinach is wilted and lentils are cooked.

4. Stir in yogurt and lemon juice. Garnish with cilantro and serve.

THIS RECIPE CONTAINS:

√ CALCIUM

√ CURCUMIN

√ LACTOFERRIN

√ PECTIN

√ PHYTATES

PHOSVITIN

√ POLYPHENOLS

√ *Bioflavonoids*

√ *Phenolic acids*

Tannins

√ OXALATES

LEGUMES & GRAINS

LENTIL BOLOGNESE

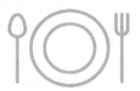

PREP TIME	COOK TIME	SERVES
15 MINUTES	20 MINUTES	6

INGREDENTS

1 cup red lentils, soaked overnight

1 cup sliced white mushrooms

3 medium carrots, finely-diced

1 medium onion, chopped

3 cloves garlic, minced

2 cups tomato sauce

1/3 cup chopped fresh basil

1/3 cup chopped fresh parsley

1/4 cup half and half

1/4 cup sunflower seeds

3 tablespoons avocado oil

1 tablespoon chili powder

salt to taste

DIRECTIONS

1. Use a food processor to blend mushroom and sunflower seeds into rice-size. Set aside. Then blend soaked lentils until tiny pieces. Add to the lentils.

2. In a pan, add oil and sauté garlic, carrot and onion until fragrant.

3. Add the lentil mixture. Sauté for 2-3 minutes. Add tomato sauce and simmer for 8-10 minutes or until lentils are cooked.

4. Stir in the rest of the ingredients. Season with salt and pepper.

THIS RECIPE CONTAINS:

√ CALCIUM	√ POLYPHENOLS
CURCUMIN	√ *Bioflavonoids*
√ LACTOFERRIN	√ *Phenolic acids*
√ PECTIN	*Tannins*
√ PHYTATES	√ OXALATES
PHOSVITIN	

LEGUMES & GRAINS

EASY LENTIL CURRY

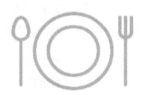

PREP TIME	COOK TIME	SERVES
5 MINUTES	35 MINUTES	4

INGREDENTS

1 1/2 cups red lentils

1 medium onion, diced

1 large carrot, diced

3 1/2 cup vegetable broth

1/2 cup coconut cream

1 1/2 tablespoons coconut oil

1 tablespoon curry powder

1 teaspoon ground ginger

1/2 teaspoon turmeric

salt and pepper to taste

DIRECTIONS

1. In a pan, add oil and sauté onion and carrots with all spices until fragrant. Add lentils and stir fry for 1 minutes. Add broth and simmer for 25-30 minutes or until lentils are cooked.

2. Stir in coconut milk. Season with salt and pepper. Serve immediately.

THIS RECIPE CONTAINS:

√ CALCIUM   √ POLYPHENOLS

√ CURCUMIN   √ Bioflavonoids

LACTOFERRIN   √ Phenolic acids

√ PECTIN   Tannins

√ PHYTATES   √ OXALATES

PHOSVITIN

LEGUMES & GRAINS

CHEESY BROCCOLI BROWN RICE

PREP TIME
10 MINUTES

COOK TIME
35 MINUTES

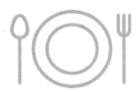

SERVES
4

INGREDENTS

1 cup uncooked brown rice

1 medium broccoli, florets only, finely chopped

2 cups shredded cheddar cheese

2 cups vegetable broth

1/2 medium onion, chopped

2 cloves garlic, minced

1 tablespoon coconut oil

salt and pepper to taste

DIRECTIONS

1. In a pan, add oil and sauté garlic and onion until fragrant. Add rice and stir fry for 1 minutes. Add broth and simmer for 25-30 minutes.

2. Add the broccoli on top of the rice. Cook covered for another 5 minutes.

3. Remove from heat. Stir in cheese. Season with salt and pepper. Serve immediately.

THIS RECIPE CONTAINS:

√ CALCIUM   √ POLYPHENOLS

CURCUMIN   √ *Bioflavonoids*

√ LACTOFERRIN   √ *Phenolic acids*

√ PECTIN   *Tannins*

√ PHYTATES   √ OXALATES

PHOSVITIN

LEGUMES & GRAINS

MEXICAN BROWN RICE

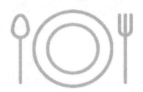

PREP TIME	COOK TIME	SERVES
10 MINUTES	40 MINUTES	4

INGREDENTS

1 cup uncooked brown rice, rinsed

1 15-ounce can black beans, rinsed and drained

4 medium tomatoes, chopped

2 cloves garlic

1 medium onion, chopped

1 1/4 cups vegetable broth

1/4 cup chopped fresh parsley

1 tablespoon avocado oil

2 teaspoons Mexican chili powder

1 teaspoon curry powder

1/2 teaspoon turmeric

salt and pepper to taste

DIRECTIONS

1. Soak the brown rice with water and set aside.

2. In a pan, add oil and sauté garlic and onion until fragrant. Add tometoes and all seasoning. Cook until tomatoes are tender.

3. Add broth and drained rice. Simmer for 20 minutes. Add beans and simmer for another 20 minutes. Season with salt and pepper. Garnish with fresh parsley and serve.

THIS RECIPE CONTAINS:

CALCIUM	√ POLYPHENOLS
√ CURCUMIN	√ Bioflavonoids
LACTOFERRIN	√ Phenolic acids
√ PECTIN	Tannins
√ PHYTATES	√ OXALATES
PHOSVITIN	

LEGUMES & GRAINS

BUTTERNUT SQUASH SPELT RISOTTO

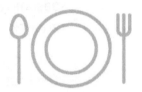

PREP TIME
15 MINUTES

COOK TIME
45 MINUTES

SERVES
4

INGREDENTS

1 medium butternut squash, seeded and cut into chunks

1 1/4 cup pearled spelt

3 cups vegetable broth

2 cups baby spinach

2/3 cup dry white wine

1/2 cup pine nuts

1/2 cup grated parmesan cheese

3 tablespoons avocado oil

3 tablespoons butter

4 shallots, chopped

4 cloves garlic, minced

8 sage leaves, chopped

salt and pepper to taste

DIRECTIONS

1. Preheat the oven to 375 °F.

2. Toss butternut squash with avocado oil, garlic and sage. Season with salt and pepper. Roast for 25-30 minutes until tender.

3. In a pan, sauté shallot with butter until tender. Add spelt and stir fry for about 1 minute. Add wine. Cook while stirring until the moisture is mostly absorbed.

4. Add broth in batches, each time cook until the liquid is absorbed. Cook until spelt is tender.

5. Stir in roasted squash, pine nuts and spinach. Season with salt and pepper. Cook until heat thoroughly.

6. Top with grated cheese and serve.

THIS RECIPE CONTAINS:

√ CALCIUM

CURCUMIN

√ LACTOFERRIN

√ PECTIN

√ PHYTATES

PHOSVITIN

√ POLYPHENOLS

√ Bioflavonoids

√ Phenolic acids

Tannins

√ OXALATES

LEGUMES & GRAINS

MUSHROOM AND THYME
BROWN RICE

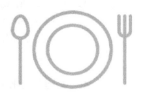

PREP TIME	COOK TIME	SERVES
10 MINUTES	50 MINUTES	4

INGREDENTS

1 cup uncooked brown rice

8 ounces cremini mushrooms, sliced

1/2 medium onion, chopped

2 cloves garlic

2 cups vegetable broth

1/4 cup grated parmesan cheese

3 tablespoons minced fresh parsley

1 tablespoon minced fresh thyme

1 1/2 tablespoons avocado oil

salt and pepper to taste

DIRECTIONS

1. In a pan, add 1/2 tablespoon of oil and sauté mushrooms with thyme until soften. Set aside.

2. Add the rest of the oil and sauté garlic and onion until fragrant. Add rice and stir fry for 1 minutes. Add broth and simmer for 25-30 minutes or until rice softens.

3. Stir in mushrooms and parsley. Season with salt and pepper. Top with cheese and serve

THIS RECIPE CONTAINS:

√ CALCIUM   √ POLYPHENOLS

CURCUMIN   √ *Bioflavonoids*

√ LACTOFERRIN   √ *Phenolic acids*

√ PECTIN   *Tannins*

√ PHYTATES   √ OXALATES

PHOSVITIN

LEGUMES & GRAINS

CREAMY CHICKEN WILD RICE

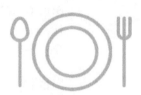

PREP TIME
10 MINUTES

COOK TIME
60 MINUTES

SERVES
6

INGREDENTS

5 cups leftover wild rice

1 small onion, chopped

4 cloves garlic, minced

1 pound skinless chicken
breast, diced

2/3 cup half and half

1/3 cup chicken broth

1/2 cup grated parmesan
cheese

1/4 cup chopped fresh
parsley

2 tablespoons avocado oil

1/4 teaspoon dried
oregano

1/4 teaspoon dried thyme

1/4 teaspoon dries parsley

salt and pepper to taste

DIRECTIONS

1. In a pan, add oil and sauté garlic and onion until fragrant. Add chicken and herbs. Season with salt and pepper. Cooked for about 5 minutes or until chicken is cooked through.

2. Add rice, half and half and broth. Bring to a boil and simmer until thickened.

3. Stir in cheese and heat on low until cheese melts. Adjust seasoning if needed. Garnish with fresh parsley and serve.

THIS RECIPE CONTAINS:

√ CALCIUM

CURCUMIN

√ LACTOFERRIN

√ PECTIN

√ PHYTATES

PHOSVITIN

√ POLYPHENOLS

√ Bioflavonoids

√ Phenolic acids

Tannins

√ OXALATES

FISH & CHICKEN

LENTIL CHICKEN SAUSAGES

PREP TIME
5 MINUTES

COOK TIME
10 MINUTES

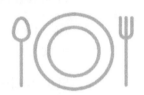

SERVES
6

INGREDENTS

12 ounces lean ground chicken

2 large eggs, whites only

1 cup chopped onion

1/2 cup dry red lentils

1/4 cup mozzarella cheese

1/4 cup parmesan cheese

6 tablespoons whole-wheat breadcrumbs

2 tablespoons flax seed meal

2 tablespoons avocado oil

1/2 teaspoon salt

1/4 teaspoon pepper

DIRECTIONS

1. In a small bowl, mix the flaxseed meal and egg white. Set aside.

2. In a medium pot, add lentil and cover with water by 1-inch. Bring it to boil and cook for 15 minutes. Drain the lentils and mash well.

3. In a large bowl, combine all ingredients.

4. Divide the mixture into 12 portions and shape into patties.

5. Spray a non-stick pan. Heat the patties for 3-5 minutes over low/medium heat until brown. Flip and heat for another 3-5 minutes.

THIS RECIPE CONTAINS:

√ CALCIUM	√ POLYPHENOLS
CURCUMIN	√ *Bioflavonoids*
√ LACTOFERRIN	√ *Phenolic acids*
√ PECTIN	*Tannins*
√ PHYTATES	OXALATES
√ PHOSVITIN	

FISH & CHICKEN

CHICKEN FAJITA

PREP TIME
10 MINUTES

COOK TIME
10 MINUTES

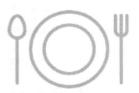

SERVES
4

INGREDENTS

1 pound skinless chicken breast, sliced

1 green bell pepper, cut into strips

1 small onion, cut into strips

2 cloves garlic, minced

1 tablespoon lemon juice

1 teaspoon ground coriander

1 teaspoon dried oregano

1/2 teaspoon ground ginger

1/2 teaspoon turmeric

1/2 teaspoon paprika

1/4 teaspoon salt

1/4 teaspoon pepper

DIRECTIONS

1. Sauté chicken with salt and pepper until cooked through. Then add onion, bell peppers and sauté until soft.

2. Add lemon juice, all herbs and spices. Sauté for another 2 minutes. Serve immediately.

THIS RECIPE CONTAINS:

CALCIUM	√ POLYPHENOLS
√ CURCUMIN	√ *Bioflavonoids*
LACTOFERRIN	√ *Phenolic acids*
PECTIN	*Tannins*
PHYTATES	OXALATES
PHOSVITIN	

FISH & CHICKEN

CHEESY SPICY HALIBUT

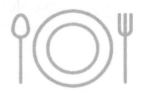

PREP TIME	COOK TIME	SERVES
15 MINUTES	10 MINUTES	2

INGREDENTS

1/2 pound skinless halibut fillets

2 medium tomatoes, chopped

1 green onion, chopped

1/4 cup parmesan cheese

1 tablespoon avocado oil

2 teaspoons mayonnaise

1/2 tablespoons lemon juice

1/2 teaspoon hot sauce

1/8 teaspoon salt

DIRECTIONS

1. Preheat the oven to 425°F.

2. In a medium bowl, combine all ingredients except fish.

3. Season the fish with salt and pepper. Place the fish on a baking dish. Bake for 10 minutes.

4. Spread the cheese mixture on top and bake for another 5 minutes or until cheese are bubbly and golden brown.

THIS RECIPE CONTAINS:

√ CALCIUM

CURCUMIN

√ LACTOFERRIN

√ PECTIN

PHYTATES

PHOSVITIN

√ POLYPHENOLS

√ Bioflavonoids

√ Phenolic acids

Tannins

√ OXALATES

FISH & CHICKEN

SALMON IN CREAMED SPINACH

PREP TIME
10 MINUTES

COOK TIME
15 MINUTES

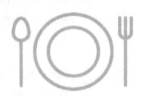

SERVES
4

INGREDENTS

4 wild caught salmon fillet, 4-6 ounces each

2 cups half and half

1 cup heavy cream

1 large bunch spinach

1/2 cup chopped fresh dill

1/4 cup chopped fresh parsley

2 tablespoons avocado oil

1 tablespoon lemon juice

1 teaspoon salt

DIRECTIONS

1. Broil the salmon for about 5 minutes. Break into chunks and set aside to cool.

2. In a sauce pan, add all ingredients except lemon juice. Cook over medium heat until spinach are soft,about 8-10 minutes. Stir in lemon juice.

3. Use a food processor or blender to blend the sauce in small batches.

4. Transfer the creamed spinach to 4 serving bowls. Top with salmon chunks and serve.

THIS RECIPE CONTAINS:

√ CALCIUM	√ POLYPHENOLS
CURCUMIN	√ Bioflavonoids
√ LACTOFERRIN	√ Phenolic acids
PECTIN	Tannins
PHYTATES	√ OXALATES
PHOSVITIN	

FISH & CHICKEN

CHICKEN PICCATA

PREP TIME
5 MINUTES

COOK TIME
20 MINUTES

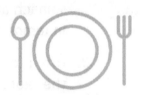

SERVES
4

INGREDENTS

4 skinless chicken breasts

1 1/2 cup chicken broth

2 lemons, juice only

1/4 cup chopped fresh parsley

2 tablespoons butter

2 tablespoons heavy cream

salt to taste

DIRECTIONS

1. In a pan, add butter. Brown the chicken breast, about 3 minutes per side. Season with salt. Let it cool and cut into chunks

2. Add the rest of the ingredients. Bring to a boil and then reduce to low. Simmer for 10 minutes.

3. Add chicken and heat until hot thoroughly.

THIS RECIPE CONTAINS:

√ CALCIUM

CURCUMIN

√ LACTOFERRIN

PECTIN

PHYTATES

PHOSVITIN

POLYPHENOLS

Bioflavonoids

Phenolic acids

Tannins

√ OXALATES

FISH & CHICKEN

CREAMY TURMRIC COD

PREP TIME
5 MINUTES

COOK TIME
20 MINUTES

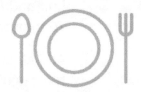

SERVES
3

INGREDENTS

3 cod fillets

1/2 cup heavy cream

1/2 teaspoon ground turmeric

2 tablespoons chopped fresh parsley

1/2 teaspoon salt

DIRECTIONS

1. Preheat the oven to 350 °F.

2. In a small bowl, combine coconut milk, turmeric and salt.

3. Line the cod fillets on a baking dish. Pour the coconut mixture onto and sprinkle with parsley. Bake for 15-20 minutes or until cod is cooked through.

THIS RECIPE CONTAINS:

√ CALCIUM

√ CURCUMIN

√ LACTOFERRIN

PECTIN

PHYTATES

PHOSVITIN

√ POLYPHENOLS

√ *Bioflavonoids*

Phenolic acids

Tannins

√ OXALATES

FISH & CHICKEN

WHITE BEAN AND CHICKEN SOUP

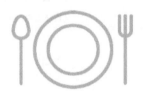

PREP TIME	COOK TIME	SERVES
10 MINUTES	20 MINUTES	6

INGREDENTS

1 pound skinless chicken breast, diced

1 leek, chopped

1 small onion, chopped

1 can 15-ounce cannellini beans, rinsed and drained

2 cups chicken broth

1 tablespoon coconut oil

1 tablespoon chopped fresh sage

1 tablespoon chopped fresh dill

1 teaspoon chopped fresh rosemary

1 bay leave

1/4 teaspoon salt

DIRECTIONS

1. Spray a large pot. Sauté leek and onion over medium heat until softened.

2. Add broth and 2 cups of water. Bring it to a boil. Then add all other ingredients. Heat for 5-10 minutes.

THIS RECIPE CONTAINS:

CALCIUM

CURCUMIN

LACTOFERRIN

√ PECTIN

√ PHYTATES

PHOSVITIN

√ POLYPHENOLS

√ Bioflavonoids

√ Phenolic acids

Tannins

√ OXALATES

FISH & CHICKEN

CHICKEN SATAY

PREP TIME
10 MINUTES

COOK TIME
20 MINUTES

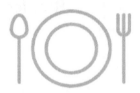

SERVES
6

INGREDENTS

1 pound chicken breast, diced

1 cup heavy cream

2 cloves garlic, minced

1/4 cup peanut butter

1 tablespoon maple syrup

1 teaspoon turmeric

1/4 teaspoon salt

DIRECTIONS

1. Preheat broiler.

2. Thread the chicken onto 12 skewers.

3. In a small bowl, combine all other ingredients. Coat the skewer with the half of the sauce. Set aside to marinade for 10 minutes. Then broil for 10-15 minutes or until crispy.

4. While the meat is broiling, heat the remaining sauce in a pan. Pour over the skewer and serve.

THIS RECIPE CONTAINS:

√ CALCIUM

√ CURCUMIN

√ LACTOFERRIN

√ PECTIN

PHYTATES

√ PHOSVITIN

√ POLYPHENOLS

√ *Bioflavonoids*

√ *Phenolic acids*

Tannins

√ OXALATES

FISH & CHICKEN

SPINACH FETA STUFFED CHICKEN

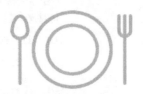

PREP TIME	COOK TIME	SERVES
10 MINUTES	25 MINUTES	2

INGREDENTS

2 boneless, skinless chicken breast, flattened

5 ounces frozen spinach, thawed and squeeze

1/4 cup feta cheese

3 tablespoons ricotta cheese

2 tablespoons chopped green onion

2 tablespoons chopped fresh parsley

1/2 tablespoon fresh dill

1 clove garlic

salt and pepper to taste

DIRECTIONS

1. Preheat the oven to 350°F.

2. Sauté the green onion and garlic until fragrant. Add spinach, parsley and dill. Cool until heated through. Season with salt and pepper.

3. Remove from heat and stir in feta cheese and ricotta cheese.

4. Divide the mixture onto the chicken breast. Roll up. Rub the chicken with salt and pepper.

5. Bake for 25 minutes.

THIS RECIPE CONTAINS:

√ CALCIUM   √ POLYPHENOLS

CURCUMIN   √ *Bioflavonoids*

√ LACTOFERRIN   √ *Phenolic acids*

PECTIN   *Tannins*

PHYTATES   √ OXALATES

PHOSVITIN

FISH & CHICKEN

POMODORO CHICKEN
WITH SQUASH

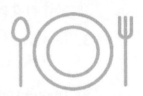

PREP TIME
20 MINUTES

COOK TIME
20 MINUTES

SERVES
4

INGREDENTS

1/2 medium butternut
squash, seeded and
spiralized

12 ounces boneless
skinless chicken breast,
diced

1 can 14.5-ounce crushed
tomatoes

1/2 cup chopped onion

1 clove garlic, minced

1 1/2 tablespoons chopped
basil

salt and pepper to taste

DIRECTIONS

1. In a pan, brown the chicken. Season with salt and pepper. Then add garlic and onion sauté for 2 minutes.

2. Stir in tomatoes and bring the mixture to a boil. Reduce to low heat and simmer for 5-10 minutes to reduce.

3. Toss in squash noodles and heat for 3-4 minutes or until the desired texture is reached. Sprinkle with basil and serve.

THIS RECIPE CONTAINS:

CALCIUM	√ POLYPHENOLS
CURCUMIN	√ *Bioflavonoids*
LACTOFERRIN	√ *Phenolic acids*
√ PECTIN	*Tannins*
PHYTATES	OXALATES
PHOSVITIN	

FISH & CHICKEN

CHICKEN BASQUE

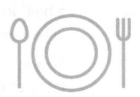

PREP TIME	COOK TIME	SERVES
20 MINUTES	20 MINUTES	2

INGREDENTS

1 medium zucchini, spiralized

2 skinless chicken breast, diced

1/2 cup grape tomatoes, quartered

1/4 cup thinly sliced red bell peppers

1/4 cup chopped yellow onion

1/4 cup chicken broth

1 tablespoon coconut oil

1 tablespoon chopped fresh parsley

1/4 teaspoon fresh thyme

1/8 teaspoon paprika

1/8 teaspoon red pepper flakes

1/8 teaspoon salt

DIRECTIONS

1. In a pan, add oil and sauté chicken with salt until cooked through. Then add paprika, bell peppers and onion sauté for 2 minutes.

2. Add tomatoes, broth, thyme, red pepper flakes and bring the mixture to a boil. Reduce to low heat and simmer for 5-10 minutes to reduce.

3. Toss in zoodles and heat for 2-3 minutes or until the desired texture is reached. Sprinkle with parsley and serve.

THIS RECIPE CONTAINS:

CALCIUM	√ POLYPHENOLS
CURCUMIN	√ *Bioflavonoids*
LACTOFERRIN	√ *Phenolic acids*
√ PECTIN	*Tannins*
PHYTATES	√ OXALATES
PHOSVITIN	

FISH & CHICKEN

SPAGHETTI SQUASH CHICKEN

ALFREDO

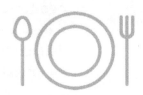

PREP TIME	COOK TIME	SERVES
60 MINUTES	20 MINUTES	4

INGREDENTS

1 small spaghetti squash, halved

2 skinless chicken breast, cooked and diced

1 medium zucchini, peeled and diced

1 tablespoon coconut oil

For the sauce:

1/4 cup coconut oil

1 1/4 cups grated parmesan cheese

1 cup heavy cream

2 tablespoons chopped fresh basil

2 tablespoons chopped fresh parsley

1/2 teaspoon oregano

1/2 teaspoon nutmeg

salt and pepper to taste

DIRECTIONS

1. Preheat the oven to 425 °F.

2. Put the spaghetti squash face down on a baking dish. Bake for 45 minutes. Remove the seeds and scrap out the flesh into a large bowl.

3. In a large skillet, brown the chicken. Set aside.

4. Sauté zucchini for 5 minutes. Set Aside.

5. Add all the sauce ingredients except parsley and cheese. Simmer for 5 minutes before stirring in cheese quickly.

6. Add the spaghetti squash, chicken, zucchini back. Heat for another 1-2 minutes. Add parsley and serve.

THIS RECIPE CONTAINS:

√ CALCIUM	√ POLYPHENOLS
CURCUMIN	√ Bioflavonoids
√ LACTOFERRIN	Phenolic acids
√ PECTIN	Tannins
PHYTATES	√ OXALATES
PHOSVITIN	

FISH & CHICKEN

CHICKEN BIRYANI

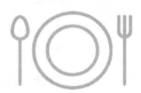

PREP TIME
2 HOURS

COOK TIME
20 MINUTES

SERVES
4

INGREDENTS

4 skinless chicken breasts, cut into bite-size

1 cup heavy cream

1 cinnamon stick

1/2 bunch coriander leaves, chopped

1 tablespoon grated fresh ginger

1 tablespoon lemon juice

1 tablespoon garam masala

1/2 teaspoon turmeric

salt to taste

DIRECTIONS

1. In a large bowl, combine all ingredients except chicken. Season with salt to taste.

2. Mix sauce with chicken thoroughly. Refrigerate for 2 hours to marinate.

3. Preheat the broiler. Line the chicken on a baking dish. Pour the marinate on top. Broil for 15-20 minutes or until chicken is cooked through.

THIS RECIPE CONTAINS:

√ CALCIUM	POLYPHENOLS
√ CURCUMIN	*Bioflavonoids*
√ LACTOFERRIN	*Phenolic acids*
PECTIN	*Tannins*
PHYTATES	OXALATES
PHOSVITIN	

FISH & CHICKEN

CHICKEN SHAWARMA

PREP TIME

2 HOURS

COOK TIME

20 MINUTES

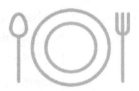

SERVES

4

INGREDENTS

4 skinless chicken breasts, cut into bite-size

4 medium tomatoes, diced

1 medium cucumber, diced

For the Marinade:

1/4 cup avocado oil

2 teaspoon ground ginger

1 teaspoon salt

3/4 teaspoon turmeric

1/4 teaspoon cinnamon

For the Sauce:

1 cup Greek yogurt

1 clove garlic, minced

1 tablespoon lemon juice

salt and pepper to taste

DIRECTIONS

1. In a large bowl, combine all ingredients except chicken. Season with salt to taste.

2. Mix sauce with chicken thoroughly. Refrigerate for 2 hours to marinate.

3. Preheat the broiler. Line the chicken on a baking dish. Pour the marinate on top. Broil for 15-20 minutes or until chicken is cooked through.

4. Serve with tomatoes, cucumber and yogurt sauce.

THIS RECIPE CONTAINS:

√ CALCIUM

√ CURCUMIN

√ LACTOFERRIN

√ PECTIN

PHYTATES

PHOSVITIN

√ POLYPHENOLS

√ *Bioflavonoids*

√ *Phenolic acids*

Tannins

√ OXALATES

FISH & CHICKEN

SALSA CHICKEN

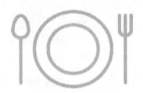

PREP TIME	COOK TIME	SERVES
2 HOURS	20 MINUTES	4

INGREDENTS

1 pound chicken tender

1 cup sour cream

For the salsa:

6 large tomatoes, chopped

1 onion, chopped

1 lime, juice only

1/2 cup green chili peppers, chopped

1 bunch cilantro, chopped

1 teaspoon salt

DIRECTIONS

1. Use a food processor to blend the salsa ingredients. Adjust seasoning if needed

2. Mix sauce with chicken thoroughly. Refrigerate for 2 hours to marinate.

3. Preheat the broiler. Line the chicken on a baking dish. Pour the marinate on top. Broil for 15-20 minutes.

4. Shred the chicken and stir in sour cream.

THIS RECIPE CONTAINS:

√ CALCIUM   √ POLYPHENOLS

CURCUMIN   √ *Bioflavonoids*

√ LACTOFERRIN   √ *Phenolic acids*

√ PECTIN   *Tannins*

PHYTATES   √ OXALATES

PHOSVITIN

FISH & CHICKEN

GEFILTE FISH

PREP TIME
2 HOURS

COOK TIME
20 MINUTES

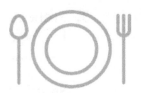

SERVES
8

INGREDENTS

1 pound halibut fillets, cut into small chunks

1/2 pound salmon fillets, cut into small chunks

3 medium carrots, peeled and grated

2 large eggs

1/2 cup chopped fresh parsley

1/4 cup chopped fresh dill

2 tablespoons avocado oil

1 tablespoon lemon juice

1 teaspoon salt

DIRECTIONS

1. Use a food processor to pulse the fish until finely ground. Add the rest of the ingredients until combined. Refrigerate the mixture for 2 hours.

2. Prepare a pot of water and bring it to a boil. Scoop spoonful of mixture. Shape into balls and put into boiling water. Cook for 15-20 minutes.

THIS RECIPE CONTAINS:

CALCIUM	√ POLYPHENOLS
CURCUMIN	√ *Bioflavonoids*
LACTOFERRIN	√ *Phenolic acids*
√ PECTIN	*Tannins*
PHYTATES	√ OXALATES
√ PHOSVITIN	

DESSERT & BEVERAGE

GOLDEN FRAPPÉ

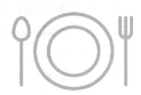

PREP TIME	COOK TIME	SERVES
2 MINUTES	NA	2

INGREDENTS

1 cup ice

4 dates, pitted and chopped

1 cup milk

1 tablespoon fresh turmeric or 1 teaspoon dried turmeric

1/2 teaspoon ground ginger

DIRECTIONS

1. Blend all ingredients on high until smooth.

THIS RECIPE CONTAINS:

√ CALCIUM	POLYPHENOLS
√ CURCUMIN	*Bioflavonoids*
√ LACTOFERRIN	*Phenolic acids*
PECTIN	*Tannins*
PHYTATES	OXALATES
PHOSVITIN	

DESSERT & BEVERAGE

VANILLA MATCHA LATTE

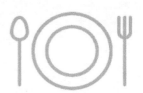

PREP TIME
2 MINUTES

COOK TIME
NA

SERVES
1

INGREDENTS

1 cup milk

4 ice cubes

1 tablespoon hot water

1 teaspoon Matcha powder

1 tablespoon maple syrup

DIRECTIONS

1. In a small bowl, dissolve Matcha powder in hot water and mix in maple syrup.

2. Blend all ingredients on high until smooth.

THIS RECIPE CONTAINS:

√ CALCIUM

CURCUMIN

√ LACTOFERRIN

PECTIN

PHYTATES

PHOSVITIN

√ POLYPHENOLS

√ *Bioflavonoids*

√ *Phenolic acids*

√ *Tannins*

OXALATES

DESSERT & BEVERAGE

AVOCADO GREEN TEA SHAKE

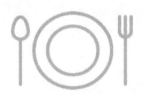

PREP TIME	COOK TIME	SERVES
2 MINUTES	NA	2

INGREDENTS

1/2 medium avocado

1/2 cup Greek yogurt

1 cup milk

1-2 tablespoons maple syrup

1 tablespoon hot water

1 teaspoon Matcha powder

DIRECTIONS

1. In a small bowl, dissolve Matcha powder in hot water and mix in maple syrup.

2. Blend all ingredients on high until smooth.

THIS RECIPE CONTAINS:

√ CALCIUM

CURCUMIN

√ LACTOFERRIN

PECTIN

PHYTATES

PHOSVITIN

√ POLYPHENOLS

√ *Bioflavonoids*

√ *Phenolic acids*

√ *Tannins*

OXALATES

DESSERT & BEVERAGE

BEET POWER JUICE

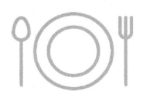

PREP TIME	COOK TIME	SERVES
5 MINUTES	NA	1

INGREDENTS

1 apple, cored and diced

1/2 cucumber, diced

1 small beetroot, peeled and diced

1/2-inch fresh ginger, peeled

1 teaspoon turmeric

1/2 teaspoon lemon juice

DIRECTIONS

1. Put the first 5 ingredients in a juicer and juice it.

2. Add lemon juice and serve

THIS RECIPE CONTAINS:

CALCIUM

√ CURCUMIN

LACTOFERRIN

√ PECTIN

PHYTATES

PHOSVITIN

√ POLYPHENOLS

√ *Bioflavonoids*

√ *Phenolic acids*

Tannins

√ OXALATES

DESSERT & BEVERAGE
PEANUT BUTTER
CHIA PUDDING

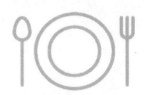

PREP TIME	COOK TIME	SERVES
20 MINUTES	NA	4

INGREDENTS

2 cups milk

1/2 cup chia seeds

1/4 cup peanut butter

1 teaspoon vanilla extract

1/4 cup honey

Pinch of salt

DIRECTIONS

1. In a mixing bowl, combine all ingredients. Divide into 4 serving bowl.

2. Refrigerate for 10 minutes. Stir before serving.

THIS RECIPE CONTAINS:

√ CALCIUM   √ POLYPHENOLS

CURCUMIN   √ *Bioflavonoids*

√ LACTOFERRIN   √ *Phenolic acids*

PECTIN   *Tannins*

√ PHYTATES   √OXALATES

PHOSVITIN

DESSERT & BEVERAGE

EASY COFFEE MOUSSE

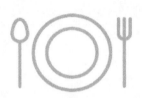

PREP TIME
135 MINUTES

COOK TIME
NA

SERVES
4

INGREDENTS

1 cup ricotta cheese

1/2 cup heavy cream

1/4 cup hot brewed coffee

2 tablespoons chopped almonds

1 tablespoon maple syrup

1 teaspoon gelatin powder

1/2 teaspoon instant expresso

1/2 teaspoon vanilla extract

Pinch of salt

DIRECTIONS

1. Dissolve gelatin in hot coffee. Set aside to cool.

2. Blend ricotta, expresso, vanilla extract, maple syrup and cooled coffee until smooth.

3. Add heavy cream and blend on high until whipped. Adjust sweetness if needed.

4. Divide into 4 serving bowl.

5. Refrigerate for 2 hours. Top with chopped almonds before serving.

THIS RECIPE CONTAINS:

√ CALCIUM

CURCUMIN

√ LACTOFERRIN

PECTIN

√ PHYTATES

PHOSVITIN

√ POLYPHENOLS

√ *Bioflavonoids*

√ *Phenolic acids*

√ *Tannins*

OXALATES

DESSERT & BEVERAGE

EASY CHEESY PUMPKIN PIE

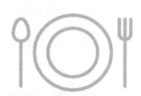

PREP TIME
500 MINUTES

COOK TIME
NA

SERVES
12

INGREDENTS

For the Crust:

3/4 cup blanched almond flour

1/2 cup flaxseed meal

1/4 cup coconut oil

2 tablespoons honey or maple syrup

1 teaspoon pumpkin pie spice

1/4 teaspoon salt

For the Filling:

4 ounces cream cheese, softened

1/3 cup pumpkin puree

1/4 cup heavy cream

2 tablespoons sour cream

3 tablespoons coconut oil

1/4 cup honey or maple syrup

DIRECTIONS

1. In a mixing bowl, combine all crust ingredients. Transfer the crust ingredients into a 9" pie pan. Mold into crust.

2. Use a food processor or blender to combine all filling ingredients. Adjust sweetness if needed.

3. Pour the filling over the crust. Refrigerate for at least 4 hours before serving.

THIS RECIPE CONTAINS:

√ CALCIUM   √ POLYPHENOLS

CURCUMIN   √ Bioflavonoids

√ LACTOFERRIN   √ Phenolic acids

PECTIN   Tannins

√ PHYTATES   √ OXALATES

PHOSVITIN

DESSERT & BEVERAGE

BLACK TEA LATTE POPSICLE

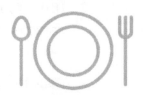

PREP TIME	COOK TIME	SERVES
500 MINUTES	NA	10

INGREDENTS

2 bags black tea

1 1/2 cup hot water

1 1/2 cup heavy whipping cream

1 cup milk

2 tablespoons honey

DIRECTIONS

1. Steep the 2 tea bags. Set aside to cool.

2. In a mixing bowl, combine all ingredients. Divide into 10 popsicle molds.

3. Freeze for at least 4 hours before serving.

THIS RECIPE CONTAINS:

√ CALCIUM

CURCUMIN

√ LACTOFERRIN

PECTIN

PHYTATES

PHOSVITIN

√ POLYPHENOLS

√ *Bioflavonoids*

√ *Phenolic acids*

√ *Tannins*

OXALATES

Made in United States
Troutdale, OR
11/04/2024

24426893R00105